NUTRITIONAL AND LIFESTYLE STRATEGIES FOR MANAGING PROSTATE CANCER

A SIMPLE GUIDE FOR MANAGING PROSTATE CANCER AND LIVING HEALTHY

TABLE OF CONTENTS

INTRODUCTION

Cancer begins when healthy cells in the prostate change and grow out of control, forming a tumor. Tumors can be either cancerous or not at all. A cancerous tumor is malignant, meaning it can grow and spread to other parts of the body. A benign tumor means the tumor can grow but will not spread.

Prostate cancer is somewhat unusual when compared with other types of cancer. This is because many prostate tumors do not

spread quickly to other parts of the body.

Some prostate cancers grow very slowly

and may not cause symptoms or problems

for years or ever. Even when prostate

cancer has spread to other parts of the

body, it often can be managed with

treatment for a long time. So people with

prostate cancer, and even those with

advanced prostate cancer, may live with

good health and quality of life for many

years. However, if cancer cannot be well

controlled with existing treatments, it can

cause symptoms like pain and fatigue and

can sometimes lead to death. An important part of managing prostate cancer is watching for growth over time to find out if it is growing slowly or quickly. Based on the pattern of growth, your doctor can decide the best available treatment options and when to give them.

Differences in diet and lifestyle may account for the variability of prostate cancer rates in different countries. Good nutrition may reduce the incidence of prostate cancer and help reduce the risk of prostate cancer progression. There are many lifestyle studies currently being conducted to further understand how diet and prostate cancer are related.

What we do know is that better nutrition lowers the risk of cardiovascular disease, diabetes, and obesity and typically improves overall health and well-being. Approximately one-third of cancer deaths among adults in the U.S. are attributed to diet, including diet's impact on obesity. Additionally, a healthy diet helps to increase energy levels, facilitate recovery and enhance the immune system.

EATING A HEALTHY DIET

FOODS TO EAT

Cancer patients need to eat a healthy diet to support their overall health and recovery. A nutritionally balanced diet can support the body' s immune system and help with recovery. Here are a few foods cancer patients should include in their diet::

1. Fruits and vegetables are packed with vitamins, minerals and ant, and antioxidants that help fight cancer and other illnesses.

Aim for a variety of colorful fruits and vegetables, including leafy greens, berries, citrus fruits, and cruciferous vegetables like broccoli and cauliflower.

2. Whole Grains: Brown Rice, Quinoa, and Whole Wheat Bread are all sources of fiber and other essential nutrients that promote digestion and overall health.

3. Lean protein: Protein is important for building and repairing tissues in the body. Choose lean sources of protein like chicken, fish, beans, and tofu.

4. Healthy fats: Nuts, seeds, and fatty fish are all sources of healthy fats, which play an important role in reducing inflammation and promoting heart health.

5. Water: Drinking water is essential for overall health and helps to eliminate toxins from the body.

Cancer patients should also consult with their healthcare provider about dietary restrictions and recommendations based on their specific conditions and treatment plan.

Foods to Avoid

While many foods can be helpful for cancer patients, some foods should be avoided or restricted to promote overall health and wellness.

Here are some foods that you may want to avoid as a cancer patient:

1. Processed meats, such as bacon, sausage, or deli meat, are high in sodium, and preservatives, and can increase your risk of cancer. Red meat, such as beef, pork,

or lamb, should also be avoided as it can increase your body's inflammation.

2. Sugary and processed foods, such as sugar and refined carbohydrates, can cause your body to become more inflamed, which can lead to cancer. Don't eat sugary foods, candy, or baked goods.

3. Alcohol: Drinking alcohol can raise your risk of cancer in breast, liver, or colorectal cancer. It's best to limit your alcohol intake or abstain from drinking alcohol all together.

4. Fried foods and high-saturated and trans fats: Fried foods, such as fried chicken and

fried fish, are high in saturated and trans fats, which can increase inflammation in your body and lead to weight gain. Choose whole foods whenever possible, and read labels carefully.

5. Foods with preservatives and additives: Many processed foods have preservatives and additives that can be damaging to your body. Make sure to only eat whole foods and read the ingredients on the label carefully.

As with all dietary advice, cancer patients need to discuss with their healthcare provider any dietary restrictions or dietary

recommendations that may be appropriate

based on their specific needs and treatment

plan.

STAYING PHYSICALLY ACTIVE

Staying physically active is important for overall health and well-being, especially for prostate cancer patients Exercise regularly can assist preserve muscle flexibility and strength while reducing fatigue and boosting mood. Here are some recommended exercises for prostate cancer patients:

1. Aerobic exercise: Aerobic exercises like walking, jogging, cycling, and swimming can help improve cardiovascular health and endurance. On most days of the week, try

to get in at least 30 minutes of moderate-intensity aerobic activity.

2. Resistance training: Using weights or resistance bands during resistance training can assist maintain strength and muscle mass. Focus on exercises that target the major muscle groups, such as squats, lunges, and chest presses.

3. Stretching: Stretching exercises can help improve flexibility and range of motion, which can be especially important after surgery or radiation therapy. Gentle yoga or tai chi can also help improve balance and reduce stress.

4. Pelvic floor exercises: Pelvic floor exercises, also known as Kegels, can help

improve urinary incontinence and sexual function after prostate cancer treatment. The muscles that govern urine flow are contracted and relaxed during these workouts.

Prostate cancer patients need to talk to their healthcare provider before starting any exercise program, especially if they have any physical limitations or concerns. A physical therapist may also be able to guide safe and effective exercises for prostate cancer patients.

Maintaining a healthy weight

Importance of weight management

Maintaining a healthy weight is crucial for prostate cancer patients as it can improve their overall quality of life and increase their chances of successful treatment. Here are some reasons why weight management is important for prostate cancer patients:

1. Treatment effectiveness: Studies have
shown that overweight and obese men with
prostate cancer have a higher risk of
treatment failure, recurrence, and death
compared to those with a healthy weight.
This is because excess fat tissue can
promote cancer cell growth and interfere
with cancer treatments' effectiveness.

2. Side effects management: Prostate
cancer treatments such as surgery,
radiation, and hormone therapy can cause
side effects such as fatigue, nausea, and
loss of muscle mass. Maintaining a healthy

weight can help patients to better tolerate these side effects and improve their recovery after treatment.

3. Overall health: Obesity and overweight are associated with an increased risk of cardiovascular disease, diabetes, and other chronic conditions. Prostate cancer patients who maintain a healthy weight are better able to manage these conditions and reduce their risk of developing other health complications.

Developing a healthy eating and exercise plan

Developing a healthy eating and exercise plan can seem daunting, but it's essential for maintaining a healthy lifestyle. Start by setting achievable goals and creating a realistic schedule that fits your lifestyle. Incorporate a variety of nutrient-dense foods into your diet, such as whole grains, lean proteins, and colorful fruits and vegetables. Avoid processed and high-sugar foods as much as possible.

In terms of exercise, find activities that you enjoy and can commit to regularly. This could be anything from jogging to yoga to weight lifting. Aim for at least 30 minutes of moderate exercise most days of the week.

Remember to stay consistent and patient with yourself as you work towards your goals. It's important to make sustainable lifestyle changes rather than quick-fix solutions. Your fitness and health goals are attainable if you put effort and persistence into them.

Limiting alcohol consumption

The Link between alcohol and prostate cancer

Limiting alcohol consumption is beneficial in reducing the risk of prostate cancer. Prostate cancer is a common type of cancer that affects men, with over 160,000 new cases diagnosed in the United

States each year. While various factors can increase the risk of prostate cancer, including age, family history, and race, lifestyle choices such as alcohol consumption can also play a role.

Studies have shown that excessive alcohol consumption can increase the risk of developing prostate cancer. This is because alcohol can damage DNA and other cells in the body, leading to mutations and abnormal growth. Additionally, alcohol can interfere with the body's ability to absorb and utilize essential nutrients that are important for prostate health.

To reduce the risk of prostate cancer, it is recommended that men limit their alcohol consumption. The American Cancer Society recommends that men have no more than two drinks per day, while the National Institute on Alcohol Abuse and Alcoholism recommends no more than four drinks per day. It is also important to note that heavy drinking, defined as more than eight drinks per week, can increase the risk of prostate cancer.

In addition to limiting alcohol consumption, other lifestyle choices can also help reduce the risk of prostate cancer. This includes maintaining a healthy diet, exercising regularly, and not smoking. Regular prostate screenings can also help detect any potential issues early on, increasing the chances of successful treatment.

Recommended alcohol intake
For prostate cancer patients, the recommended alcohol intake may differ from the general population. Studies have

shown that excessive alcohol consumption may increase the risk of prostate cancer and worsen the outcomes for those who have already been diagnosed with the disease. Therefore, it is recommended that prostate cancer patients limit their alcohol consumption or avoid it altogether.

According to the American Cancer Society, men who have been diagnosed with prostate cancer should limit their alcohol intake to no more than one drink per day. This is because excessive alcohol consumption can interfere with cancer treatment and increase the risk of complications. Additionally, alcohol can interact with certain medications used to treat prostate cancer, such as hormone therapy.

It is also important to note that some prostate cancer treatments, such as radiation therapy, may increase the risk of side effects from alcohol consumption. Therefore, prostate cancer patients need to discuss their alcohol intake with their healthcare provider and follow their recommendations.

MANAGING STRESS

Effects of chronic stress on the Body

Chronic stress can have significant effects on the body, especially for prostate cancer patients. Studies have shown that chronic stress can weaken the immune system and increase inflammation, which can worsen the outcomes for those who have already been diagnosed with the disease.

For prostate cancer patients, chronic stress can also lead to increased anxiety and depression, which can negatively impact their overall quality of life. Additionally, stress can interfere with sleep, which is important for the body's natural healing processes.

Furthermore, chronic stress can also lead to unhealthy coping mechanisms such as smoking and excessive alcohol consumption, increasing the risk of complications and worsening the outcomes for prostate cancer patients.

Therefore, prostate cancer patients need to manage their stress levels through healthy coping mechanisms such as exercise, meditation, and therapy. It is also important for healthcare providers to screen for and address any mental health concerns in prostate cancer patients to improve their overall well-being and treatment outcomes.

Chronic stress can have a significant significantly negative effect on prostate cancer patients. It is important to manage stress levels through healthy coping mechanisms and address any mental health concerns to improve treatment outcomes and overall quality of life.

Healthy stress management techniques

1. Exercise: Regular exercise can help reduce stress levels, improve mood, and boost the immune system. Prostate cancer patients should consult with their healthcare provider before starting any exercise regimen.

2. Meditation and relaxation techniques: Mindfulness meditation, deep breathing

exercises, and yoga can help reduce stress levels and improve overall well-being.

3. Therapy: Speaking with a therapist or counselor can help prostate cancer patients cope with the emotional stress of their diagnosis and treatment.

4. Support groups: Joining a support group can provide prostate cancer patients with a sense of community and support, which can help reduce stress levels.

5. Healthy lifestyle choices: Eating a balanced diet, getting enough sleep, and avoiding unhealthy coping mechanisms such as smoking and excessive alcohol consumption can all help reduce stress levels and improve overall health.

By incorporating these healthy stress management techniques into their daily routine, prostate cancer patients can improve their overall well-being and treatment outcomes. Healthcare providers need to educate patients on these techniques and provide resources for support.

TAKING SUPPLEMENT

Potential benefits of supplements for prostate cancer patients include:

1. Vitamin D: Studies have shown that vitamin D may help reduce the risk of prostate cancer progression and improve treatment outcomes.

2. Omega-3 fatty acids: Omega-3 fatty acids may help reduce inflammation and improve overall health in prostate cancer patients.

3. Green tea extract: Green tea extract contains antioxidants that may help reduce the risk of prostate cancer progression and improve treatment outcomes.

4. Selenium: Selenium is a mineral that may help reduce the risk of prostate cancer progression and improve overall health in prostate cancer patients.

5. Lycopene: Lycopene is a carotenoid found in tomatoes and other fruits and vegetables that may help reduce the risk of prostate cancer progression.

Prostate cancer patients need to speak with their healthcare provider before taking any supplements, as some may interact with medications or have negative side effects. Additionally, using supplements in place of medical care is not advised.

Prostate cancer is a common cancer that affects men, especially those above 50 years old. It is a slow-growing cancer that can be managed effectively with proper treatment and lifestyle changes. One of the lifestyle changes that patients may consider is taking supplements to improve their overall health and well-being. However, before taking any supplements, it is essential to consult with the healthcare team to ensure that they are safe and effective.

The healthcare team comprises various professionals, including doctors, nurses, dietitians, and pharmacists, who work together to provide comprehensive care for patients. They are trained to evaluate the patient's medical history, current health status, and potential risks and benefits of any treatment or supplement. Consulting with the healthcare team before taking supplements is crucial for prostate cancer patients for several reasons.

Firstly, some supplements may interact with medications used to treat prostate cancer. For instance, some supplements may interfere with hormone therapy, which is a standard treatment for prostate cancer. Hormone therapy works by reducing the levels of testosterone in the body, which can slow down the growth of cancer cells. However, some supplements may increase testosterone levels, which can counteract the effects of hormone therapy and worsen the patient's condition.

Secondly, some supplements may have adverse effects on the patient's health. For example, high doses of vitamin E supplements have been linked to an increased risk of prostate cancer. Similarly, some herbal supplements may cause allergic reactions or interact with other medications, leading to side effects such as nausea, dizziness, or diarrhea.

Thirdly, consulting with the healthcare team can help patients make informed decisions about their health. The healthcare team can provide information about the benefits and risks of different supplements and recommend those that are safe and effective for prostate cancer patients. They can also advise patients on the appropriate dosage and frequency of supplements to avoid potential harm.

CONCLUSION

In addition to medical treatments, nutritional and lifestyle strategies can play a crucial role in managing prostate cancer. Patients should aim to maintain a healthy weight, engage in regular physical activity, and consume a balanced diet rich in fruits, vegetables, whole grains, and lean proteins. They should also limit their intake of red and processed meats, saturated and Trans fats, and sugary drinks. Certain nutrients, such as vitamin D, omega-3 fatty acids, and antioxidants, may also have beneficial effects on prostate cancer. However, patients should consult with their healthcare team before taking any supplements to ensure their safety and effectiveness. Overall, adopting healthy lifestyle habits can improve the quality of life for prostate cancer patients and reduce the risk of cancer recurrence.

www.ingramcontent.com/pod-product-compliance
Lightning Source LLC
Chambersburg PA
CBHW051857250726

48659CB00006B/2258